THIS JOURNAL
Belongs To:

_____

BEFORE & *After*

WEIGHT	WEIGHT
BMI	BMI
BODY FAT	BODY FAT
MUSCLE	MUSCLE
CHEST	CHEST
WAIST	WAIST
HIPS	HIPS
THIGHS	THIGHS
CALF	CALF
BICEP	BICEP
OTHER :	OTHER :
OTHER :	OTHER :

WEIGHT LOSS *Tracker*

WEEKLY WEIGHT LOSS TRACKER

MONTHLY GOAL

_____

DATE: _____

CHEST					
WAIST					
SHOULDERS					
UPPER ARM					
FOREARM					
CALF					
WEIGHT					
TOTAL WEIGHT LOSS >>					

MONTHLY PROGRESS *Tracker*

JAN   FEB   MAR   APR   MAY   JUN   JUL   AUG   SEP   OCT   NOV   DEC

MON	TUE	WED	THU	FRI	SAT	SUN

WEIGHT LOSS MILESTONE TRACKER

CHEAT DAY TRACKER

WEEKLY DIET SUCCESS TRACKER & NOTES

15 Task Challenge

1 CREATE A KETO JOURNAL AND DOCUMENT YOUR PROGRESS

COMPLETED ☐

2 CHOOSE 7 KETO FRIENDLY RECIPES TO TRY

COMPLETED ☐

3 CREATE A WEEKLY MEAL PLANNER

COMPLETED ☐

4 LOG EVERYTHING YOU EAT IN A WEIGHT LOSS APP

COMPLETED ☐

5 PURCHASE A FOOD SCALE AND SPIRALIZER

COMPLETED ☐

6 TRY BULLET PROOF COFFEE

COMPLETED ☐

7 WEIGH YOURSELF EVERY WEEK

COMPLETED ☐

8 GO ALCOHOL FREE FOR ONE WEEK

COMPLETED ☐

9 TRY A 12-HOUR INTERMITTENT FAST

COMPLETED ☐

10 CHECK AND LOG YOUR BODY MEASUREMENTS

COMPLETED ☐

11 LIST ALL THE REASONS WHY KETO WILL WORK FOR YOU

COMPLETED ☐

12 LEARN TO MAKE FAT BOMBS

COMPLETED ☐

13 MONITOR YOUR WATER INTAKE

COMPLETED ☐

14 INCREASE YOUR HEALTHY FAT INTAKE

COMPLETED ☐

15 TEST KETONE LEVELS USING STRIPS

COMPLETED ☐

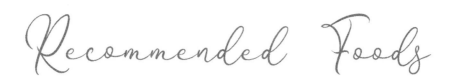
Recommended Foods

MEATS	VEGGIES	VEGGIES	FRUITS
Beef	Avocado	Cucumber	Blackberries
Sausage	Asparagus	Chards	Cranberries
Bacon	Argula	Bell Peppers	Blueberries
Lamb	Broccoli	Green Beans	Lemon
Pork	Cauliflower	Collards	Lime
Veal	Brussel Sprouts	Mushrooms	Raspberries
Chicken/Turkey	Cabbage	Spinach	Strawberries
Eggs	Celery	Olives	Plantains (paleo)

DAIRY	CONDIMENTS	OILS & FATS	HERBS & SPICES
Cheese (all kinds)	Balsamic Vinegar	Avocado Oil	Garlic
Sour Cream	Beef/Chicken Broth	Butter	Salt & Pepper
Cream Cheese	Bonito Flakes	Coconut Butter	Oregano
Heavy Cream	Tartar Sauce (keto)	Duck Fat	Paprika
Greek Yogurt	Dijon Mustard	Lard/Ghee	Cumin
Almond Milk	Mayo	Nut Oils	Chili Pepper
Cashew Milk	Low Sugar Ketchup	Olive Oil	Basil
Coconut Cream	Pickles	Pork Rinds	Ginger

BAKING	FISH/SEAFOOD	DRINKS	MISC.
Almond Flour	Anchovy	Diet Soda (moderation)	Canned Tuna
Almond Meal	Haddock / Cod	Coffee	Pesto
Cashew Flour	Halibut	Tea	Soy Sauce
Oat Fiber	Crab/Lobster	Gatorade Zero	Aioli
Psyllium Husk	Mackerel	Protein Shake	Béarnaise
Whey Protein	Salmon	Club Soda	Vinaigrette
Flax meal	Tuna	Broth	Hot Sauce
Hazelnut Flour	Red Snapper	Coconut Water	Guacamole

NOTES:

MONTH BY MONTH *Tracker*

MONTHLY WEIGHT LOSS TRACKER

JANUARY

FEBRUARY

MARCH

APRIL

MAY

JUNE

JULY

AUGUST

SEPTEMBER

OCTOBER

NOVEMBER

DECEMBER

MILESTONES

NOTES & REFLECTIONS

WEIGHT LOSS *Start Date*

Outline your most important fitness goals

Describe how you see yourself in six months

DATE	WEIGHT LOSS ACTION PLAN		PERSONAL MILESTONES
		☐	
		☐	
		☐	
		☐	
		☐	
		☐	
		☐	
		☐	
		☐	
		☐	
		☐	
		☐	

WEIGHT LOSS *Journal*

MONDAY

TUESDAY

WEDNESDAY

THURSDAY

FRIDAY

SATURDAY

SUNDAY

WEEK OF:

DATE	WEIGHT LOSS ACTION PLAN

NOTES

MY WEIGHT LOSS *Routine*

CREATING A ROUTINE FOR SUCCESS

WEIGHT LOSS SUCCESS: HABIT & ROUTINE TRACKER

DRINK LOTS OF WATER TODAY	TRACK TOTAL CARB INTAKE

COMPLETE TOP 3 GOALS OF THE DAY

1.
2.
3.

PLAN MY MEALS FOR THE DAY:

BREAKFAST	LUNCH	DINNER

DAILY TRACKER & TO DO LIST	ACCOMPLISHMENTS

NOTES

My Routine

| Morning | My Weight Loss Routine | m t w t f s s |

| Mid Day | My Weight Loss Routine | m t w t f s s |

| Evening | My Weight Loss Routine | m t w t f s s |

| Night | My Weight Loss Routine | m t w t f s s |

WEEKLY *Fasting Tracker*

Week Of: _____

MONDAY

Goal	12	1	2	3	4	5	6	7	8	9	10	11	12	1	2	3	4	5	6	7	8	9	10	11
Actual	12	1	2	3	4	5	6	7	8	9	10	11	12	1	2	3	4	5	6	7	8	9	10	11

TUESDAY

Goal	12	1	2	3	4	5	6	7	8	9	10	11	12	1	2	3	4	5	6	7	8	9	10	11
Actual	12	1	2	3	4	5	6	7	8	9	10	11	12	1	2	3	4	5	6	7	8	9	10	11

WEDNESDAY

Goal	12	1	2	3	4	5	6	7	8	9	10	11	12	1	2	3	4	5	6	7	8	9	10	11
Actual	12	1	2	3	4	5	6	7	8	9	10	11	12	1	2	3	4	5	6	7	8	9	10	11

THURSDAY

Goal	12	1	2	3	4	5	6	7	8	9	10	11	12	1	2	3	4	5	6	7	8	9	10	11
Actual	12	1	2	3	4	5	6	7	8	9	10	11	12	1	2	3	4	5	6	7	8	9	10	11

FRIDAY

Goal	12	1	2	3	4	5	6	7	8	9	10	11	12	1	2	3	4	5	6	7	8	9	10	11
Actual	12	1	2	3	4	5	6	7	8	9	10	11	12	1	2	3	4	5	6	7	8	9	10	11

SATURDAY

Goal	12	1	2	3	4	5	6	7	8	9	10	11	12	1	2	3	4	5	6	7	8	9	10	11
Actual	12	1	2	3	4	5	6	7	8	9	10	11	12	1	2	3	4	5	6	7	8	9	10	11

SUNDAY

Goal	12	1	2	3	4	5	6	7	8	9	10	11	12	1	2	3	4	5	6	7	8	9	10	11
Actual	12	1	2	3	4	5	6	7	8	9	10	11	12	1	2	3	4	5	6	7	8	9	10	11

WEEKLY *Progress*

WEEK OF : _____

Monday

Tuesday

Wednesday

Thursday

Friday

Saturday

Sunday

Notes

WEEK OF: *Meal* **LOG BOOK**

	BREAKFAST	LUNCH	DINNER	SNACKS
MONDAY				
TUESDAY				
WEDNESDAY				
THURSDAY				
FRIDAY				
SATURDAY				
SUNDAY				

MY PROGRESS *Tracker*

SLEEP TRACKER: **DATE** _____

☀ RISE: _____   ☾ BEDTIME: _____   💭 SLEEP (HRS): _____

NOTES FOR THE DAY

_____
_____
_____

IN A STATE OF KETOSIS?

YES   NO   UNSURE

WATER INTAKE TRACKER

EXERCISE / WORKOUT ROUTINE

DAILY ENERGY LEVEL		
HIGH	**MEDIUM**	**LOW**

BREAKFAST

FAT: CARBS: PROTEIN: CALORIES:

LUNCH

FAT: CARBS: PROTEIN: CALORIES:

DINNER

FAT: CARBS: PROTEIN: CALORIES:

SNACKS

FAT: CARBS: PROTEIN: CALORIES:

TOP 6 PRIORITIES OF THE DAY

END OF THE DAY TOTAL OVERVIEW

CARBS   FAT   PROTEIN   CALORIES

Macro Quick Reference

MACRO TRACKER

QTY	TYPE	PROTEIN	FAT	CARBS	CALS	NOTES

GOALS &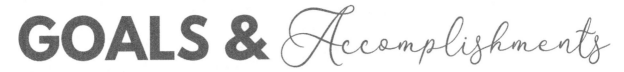

MONTH | JAN FEB MAR APR MAY JUN JUL AUG SEP OCT NOV DEC

THIS MONTH'S **GOALS**

ACTION PLAN   M T W T F S S

WEEKLY GOALS

M
T
W
T
F
S
S

NOTES:

THOUGHTS

MEALS:	BREAKFAST	LUNCH	DINNER	SNACKS
M				
T				
W				
T				
F				
S				
S				

Low Carb Grocery Ideas

FRESH PRODUCE

- Asparagus
- Avocado
- Bell Peppers
- Berries
- Broccoli
- Brussel Sprouts
- Cabbage
- Carrots
- Cauliflower
- Celery
- Cucumber
- Eggplant
- Fennel
- Garlic
- Green Beans
- Mushrooms
- Onions
- Radishes
- Salad Mix
- Squash
- Tomatoes
- Bok Choi
- Chives
- Spinach

MEAT AND SEAFOOD

- Bacon
- Beef
- Bison
- Chicken
- Deli meat
- Ground Beef / Ground Turkey
- Lamb
- Pork
- Rotisserie Chicken
- Sausage
- Turkey
- Oyster
- Fish
- Crab
- Lobster
- Scallops
- Shrimp
- Mussels

DAIRY PRODUCTS

- Butter
- Cheese
- Cream Cheese
- Eggs
- Greek Yogurt, full fat
- Heavy Whipping Cream
- Sour Cream
- Ghee
- Mayo

PANTRY ITEMS

- Avocado oil
- Beef Jerky
- Bone Broth
- Tuna, Salmon (canned)
- Coconut Butter
- Coconut Oil
- Almond Milk
- Tea/Coffee
- Pork Rinds
- Mayonnaise
- Low Carb Salad Dressing
- Olive oil, extra virgin
- Olives
- Sweeteners
- Moon Cheese
- Low Carb Protein Bars
- All Natural Peanut Butter
- Stevia
- Almonds
- Spices
- Almond Flour

FROZEN / OTHER

Low Carb Shopping List

FRESH PRODUCE

MEAT AND SEAFOOD

DAIRY PRODUCTS

PANTRY ITEMS

FROZEN / OTHER

Healthy and Friendly Foods

KETO FRIENDLY FOODS	NET CARBS	PROTEINS	FAT

FOODS TO EAT IN MODERATION	NET CARBS	PROTEINS	FAT

STAYING *On Track*

MY WEIGHT LOSS DIARY:

WATER TRACKER

LOW CARB SNACKS

NOTES & REMINDERS

DOODLE MY MOOD

BREAKFAST IDEAS

LUNCH IDEAS

DINNER IDEAS

STAYING *On Track*

MY WEIGHT LOSS DIARY:

WATER TRACKER

LOW CARB SNACKS

NOTES & REMINDERS

DOODLE MY MOOD

BREAKFAST IDEAS

LUNCH IDEAS

DINNER IDEAS

STAYING *On Track*

MY WEIGHT LOSS DIARY:

WATER TRACKER

LOW CARB SNACKS

NOTES & REMINDERS

DOODLE MY MOOD

BREAKFAST IDEAS

LUNCH IDEAS

DINNER IDEAS

STAYING *On Track*

MY WEIGHT LOSS DIARY:

WATER TRACKER

LOW CARB SNACKS

NOTES & REMINDERS

DOODLE MY MOOD

BREAKFAST IDEAS

LUNCH IDEAS

DINNER IDEAS

STAYING *On Track*

MY WEIGHT LOSS DIARY:

_____
_____
_____
_____

WATER TRACKER

NOTES & REMINDERS

DOODLE MY MOOD

LOW CARB SNACKS

BREAKFAST IDEAS

LUNCH IDEAS

DINNER IDEAS

STAYING *On Track*

MY WEIGHT LOSS DIARY:

WATER TRACKER

LOW CARB SNACKS

NOTES & REMINDERS

DOODLE MY MOOD

BREAKFAST IDEAS

LUNCH IDEAS

DINNER IDEAS

STAYING *On Track*

MY WEIGHT LOSS DIARY:

WATER TRACKER

LOW CARB SNACKS

NOTES & REMINDERS

DOODLE MY MOOD

BREAKFAST IDEAS

LUNCH IDEAS

DINNER IDEAS

MEAL *Planner*

WEEK OF

GROCERY LIST

- MON
- TUES
- WED
- THUR
- FRI
- SAT
- SUN

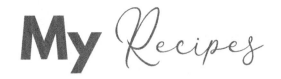

My Recipes

RECIPE NAME:

Keto	Low Carb	Paleo	Vegetarian	Vegan	Dairy Free	Gluten Free
☐	☐	☐	☐	☐	☐	☐

QTY	INGREDIENTS

RECIPE INSTRUCTIONS

NOTES & RECIPE REVIEW

Serves	
Prep Time	
Cook Time	
Tools	
Temp	

Total	Carbs	Fat	Protein	Cals

DAILY FOOD *Tracker*

FOOD TRACKER

MEAL/SNACK	NET CARBS	FAT	CAL	PROTEIN
	DAILY GOAL:			
	TOTAL:			

NOTES & MEAL IDEAS

FITNESS TRACKER

- Type
- Time
- Avg HR
- Max HR
- Reps
- Cals

Notes

DAILY OVERVIEW

- Sleep
- Water Intake
- Steps Taken
- Active Mins
- Active Hours
- Cals Burned

Notes

On Track

Goal Met

DAILY FOOD *Tracker*

FOOD TRACKER

MEAL/SNACK	NET CARBS	FAT	CAL	PROTEIN
DAILY GOAL:				
TOTAL:				

NOTES & MEAL IDEAS

FITNESS TRACKER

- Type
- Time
- Avg HR
- Max HR
- Reps
- Cals

Notes

DAILY OVERVIEW

- Sleep
- Water Intake
- Steps Taken
- Active Mins
- Active Hours
- Cals Burned

Notes

On Track

Goal Met

DAILY FOOD *Tracker*

FOOD TRACKER

MEAL/SNACK	NET CARBS	FAT	CAL	PROTEIN
DAILY GOAL:				
TOTAL:				

NOTES & MEAL IDEAS

FITNESS TRACKER

Type	
Time	
Avg HR	
Max HR	
Reps	
Cals	

Notes

DAILY OVERVIEW

Sleep	
Water Intake	
Steps Taken	
Active Mins	
Active Hours	
Cals Burned	

Notes

On Track ☐

Goal Met ☐

DAILY FOOD *Tracker*

FOOD TRACKER

MEAL/SNACK	NET CARBS	FAT	CAL	PROTEIN
DAILY GOAL:				
TOTAL:				

NOTES & MEAL IDEAS

FITNESS TRACKER

		Notes
Type		
Time		
Avg HR		
Max HR		
Reps		
Cals		

DAILY OVERVIEW

		Notes		On Track
Sleep				
Water Intake				
Steps Taken				Goal Met
Active Mins				
Active Hours				
Cals Burned				

DAILY FOOD *Tracker*

FOOD TRACKER

MEAL/SNACK	NET CARBS	FAT	CAL	PROTEIN
DAILY GOAL:				
TOTAL:				

NOTES & MEAL IDEAS

FITNESS TRACKER

- Type
- Time
- Avg HR
- Max HR
- Reps
- Cals

Notes

DAILY OVERVIEW

- Sleep
- Water Intake
- Steps Taken
- Active Mins
- Active Hours
- Cals Burned

Notes

On Track

Goal Met

DAILY FOOD *Tracker*

FOOD TRACKER

MEAL/SNACK	NET CARBS	FAT	CAL	PROTEIN
DAILY GOAL:				
TOTAL:				

NOTES & MEAL IDEAS

FITNESS TRACKER

Type	Notes
Time	
Avg HR	
Max HR	
Reps	
Cals	

DAILY OVERVIEW

Sleep	Notes	On Track ☐
Water Intake		
Steps Taken		
Active Mins		Goal Met ☐
Active Hours		
Cals Burned		

DAILY FOOD *Tracker*

FOOD TRACKER

MEAL/SNACK	NET CARBS	FAT	CAL	PROTEIN
DAILY GOAL:				
TOTAL:				

NOTES & MEAL IDEAS

FITNESS TRACKER

		Notes
Type		
Time		
Avg HR		
Max HR		
Reps		
Cals		

DAILY OVERVIEW

		Notes		
Sleep			On Track	☐
Water Intake				
Steps Taken				
Active Mins			Goal Met	☐
Active Hours				
Cals Burned				

KETO GO TO *Meals*

FAVORITE KETO FRIENDLY MEALS

BREAKFAST	LUNCH	DINNER	SNACKS
BREAKFAST	LUNCH	DINNER	SNACKS
BREAKFAST	LUNCH	DINNER	SNACKS
BREAKFAST	LUNCH	DINNER	SNACKS
BREAKFAST	LUNCH	DINNER	SNACKS
BREAKFAST	LUNCH	DINNER	SNACKS
BREAKFAST	LUNCH	DINNER	SNACKS

12 WEEK *Meal Tracker*

12 Week Challenge

MONTH	JAN	FEB	MAR	APR	MAY	JUN	JUL	AUG	SEP	OCT	NOV	DEC
WEEK	01	02	03	04	05	06	07	08	09	10	11	12

	BREAKFAST	LUNCH	DINNER	SNACKS
M				
T				
W				
T				
F				
S				
S				

GROCERY SHOPPING LIST / RECIPE INGREDIENTS

Weekly Meal Planner

Week of: _____

	Breakfast	Lunch	Dinner	Snack	Other
Monday	Carbs Fat Protein Cals TOTAL	Carbs Fat Protein Cals TOTAL	Carbs Fat Protein Cals TOTAL	Carbs Fat Protein Cals TOTAL	Carbs Fat Protein Cals TOTAL
Tuesday	Carbs Fat Protein Cals TOTAL	Carbs Fat Protein Cals TOTAL	Carbs Fat Protein Cals TOTAL	Carbs Fat Protein Cals TOTAL	Carbs Fat Protein Cals TOTAL
Wednesday	Carbs Fat Protein Cals TOTAL	Carbs Fat Protein Cals TOTAL	Carbs Fat Protein Cals TOTAL	Carbs Fat Protein Cals TOTAL	Carbs Fat Protein Cals TOTAL
Thursday	Carbs Fat Protein Cals TOTAL	Carbs Fat Protein Cals TOTAL	Carbs Fat Protein Cals TOTAL	Carbs Fat Protein Cals TOTAL	Carbs Fat Protein Cals TOTAL
Friday	Carbs Fat Protein Cals TOTAL	Carbs Fat Protein Cals TOTAL	Carbs Fat Protein Cals TOTAL	Carbs Fat Protein Cals TOTAL	Carbs Fat Protein Cals TOTAL
Saturday	Carbs Fat Protein Cals TOTAL	Carbs Fat Protein Cals TOTAL	Carbs Fat Protein Cals TOTAL	Carbs Fat Protein Cals TOTAL	Carbs Fat Protein Cals TOTAL
Sunday	Carbs Fat Protein Cals TOTAL	Carbs Fat Protein Cals TOTAL	Carbs Fat Protein Cals TOTAL	Carbs Fat Protein Cals TOTAL	Carbs Fat Protein Cals TOTAL

100 Days of Diet

STARTING WEIGHT: **DAY 100 WEIGHT:**

1	2	3	4	5	6	7	8	9	10	LBS LOST: INCHES LOST:
11	12	13	14	15	16	17	18	19	20	LBS LOST: INCHES LOST:
21	22	23	24	25	26	27	28	29	30	LBS LOST: INCHES LOST:
31	32	33	34	35	36	37	38	39	40	LBS LOST: INCHES LOST:
41	42	43	44	45	46	47	48	49	50	LBS LOST: INCHES LOST:
51	52	53	54	55	56	57	58	59	60	LBS LOST: INCHES LOST:
61	62	63	64	65	66	67	68	69	70	LBS LOST: INCHES LOST:
71	72	73	74	75	76	77	78	79	80	LBS LOST: INCHES LOST:
81	82	83	84	85	86	87	88	89	90	LBS LOST: INCHES LOST:
91	92	93	94	95	96	97	98	99	100	LBS LOST: INCHES LOST:

TOTAL WEIGHT LOST: **TOTAL INCHES LOST:**

NOTES & REFLECTIONS:

24 DAY Weight Loss Steps

WEIGHT LOSS PLAN OF ACTION:

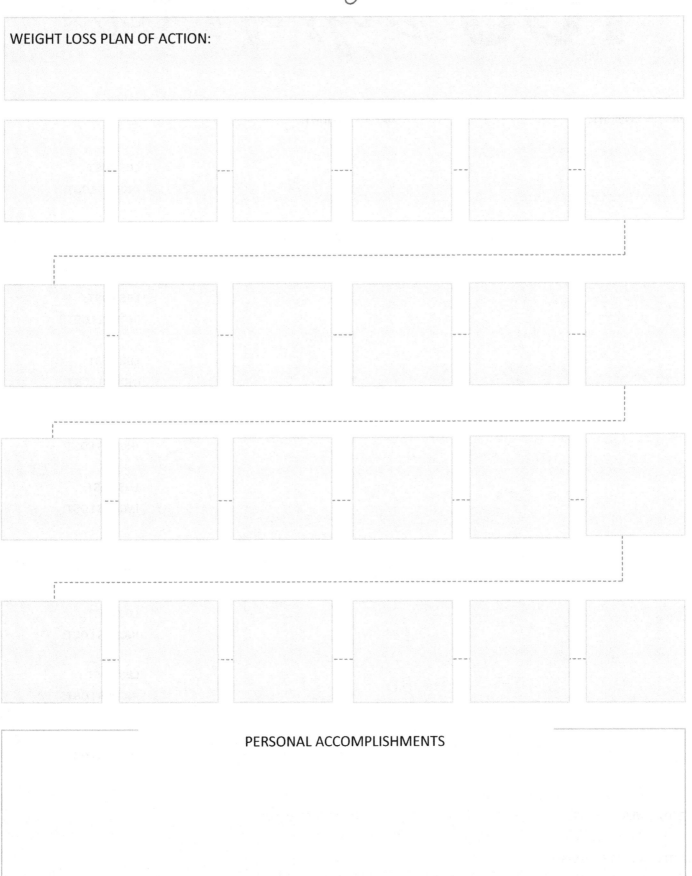

PERSONAL ACCOMPLISHMENTS

30 DAY *Diet Challenge*

WHY THIS GOAL MEANS SO MUCH

MY PLAN OF ACTION

INSPIRATIONAL REMINDERS

STARTED >

FINISHED >

1	2	3	4	5	6	7	8	9	10
11	12	13	14	15	16	17	18	19	20
21	22	23	24	25	26	27	28	29	30

30-DAY KETO RESULTS

PERSONAL ACCOMPLISHMENTS

60 Days of Diet

STARTING WEIGHT: **DAY 60 WEIGHT:**

1	2	3	4	5	6	7	8	9	10	**LBS LOST:** **INCHES LOST:**
11	12	13	14	15	16	17	18	19	20	**LBS LOST:** **INCHES LOST:**
21	22	23	24	25	26	27	28	29	30	**LBS LOST:** **INCHES LOST:**
31	32	33	34	35	36	37	38	39	40	**LBS LOST:** **INCHES LOST:**
41	42	43	44	45	46	47	48	49	50	**LBS LOST:** **INCHES LOST:**
51	52	53	54	55	56	57	58	59	60	**LBS LOST:** **INCHES LOST:**

TOTAL WEIGHT LOST: **TOTAL INCHES LOST:**

NOTES & REFLECTIONS:

30 Days of Diet

STARTING WEIGHT: **DAY 30 WEIGHT:**

| 1 | 2 | 3 | 4 | 5 | 6 | 7 | 8 | 9 | 10 |

LBS LOST:
INCHES LOST:

| 11 | 12 | 13 | 14 | 15 | 16 | 17 | 18 | 19 | 20 |

LBS LOST:
INCHES LOST:

| 21 | 22 | 23 | 24 | 25 | 26 | 27 | 28 | 29 | 30 |

LBS LOST:
INCHES LOST:

TOTAL WEIGHT LOST: **TOTAL INCHES LOST:**

NOTES:

PERSONAL ACCOMPLISHMENTS:

THOUGHTS & REFLECTIONS:

WEIGHT LOSS *Journal*

MONDAY

TUESDAY

WEDNESDAY

THURSDAY

FRIDAY

SATURDAY

SUNDAY

WEEK OF:

DATE	WEIGHT LOSS ACTION PLAN

NOTES

WEEKLY *Fasting Tracker*

Week Of: _____

MONDAY

Goal	12	1	2	3	4	5	6	7	8	9	10	11	12	1	2	3	4	5	6	7	8	9	10	11
Actual	12	1	2	3	4	5	6	7	8	9	10	11	12	1	2	3	4	5	6	7	8	9	10	11

TUESDAY

Goal	12	1	2	3	4	5	6	7	8	9	10	11	12	1	2	3	4	5	6	7	8	9	10	11
Actual	12	1	2	3	4	5	6	7	8	9	10	11	12	1	2	3	4	5	6	7	8	9	10	11

WEDNESDAY

Goal	12	1	2	3	4	5	6	7	8	9	10	11	12	1	2	3	4	5	6	7	8	9	10	11
Actual	12	1	2	3	4	5	6	7	8	9	10	11	12	1	2	3	4	5	6	7	8	9	10	11

THURSDAY

Goal	12	1	2	3	4	5	6	7	8	9	10	11	12	1	2	3	4	5	6	7	8	9	10	11
Actual	12	1	2	3	4	5	6	7	8	9	10	11	12	1	2	3	4	5	6	7	8	9	10	11

FRIDAY

Goal	12	1	2	3	4	5	6	7	8	9	10	11	12	1	2	3	4	5	6	7	8	9	10	11
Actual	12	1	2	3	4	5	6	7	8	9	10	11	12	1	2	3	4	5	6	7	8	9	10	11

SATURDAY

Goal	12	1	2	3	4	5	6	7	8	9	10	11	12	1	2	3	4	5	6	7	8	9	10	11
Actual	12	1	2	3	4	5	6	7	8	9	10	11	12	1	2	3	4	5	6	7	8	9	10	11

SUNDAY

Goal	12	1	2	3	4	5	6	7	8	9	10	11	12	1	2	3	4	5	6	7	8	9	10	11
Actual	12	1	2	3	4	5	6	7	8	9	10	11	12	1	2	3	4	5	6	7	8	9	10	11

21 DAY DIET *Challenge*

It takes just 21 days to create a healthy routine that will last a lifetime!

START DATE	END DATE

1	2	3	4	5
6	7	8	9	10
11	12	13	14	15
16	17	18	19	20
21				

NOTES
_____
_____
_____
_____
_____
_____

Grocery Inventory

DATE: _____

QTY	PRODUCE

QTY	MEAT & FISH

QTY	FROZEN FOODS

QTY	DAIRY

QTY	PANTRY

QTY	OTHER/MISC.

WEIGHT LOSS *Journal*

MONDAY

TUESDAY

WEDNESDAY

THURSDAY

FRIDAY

SATURDAY

SUNDAY

WEEK OF:

DATE	WEIGHT LOSS ACTION PLAN

NOTES

WEIGHT LOSS *Tracker*

WEEKLY WEIGHT LOSS TRACKER

MONTHLY GOAL

DATE:

CHEST					
WAIST					
SHOULDERS					
UPPER ARM					
FOREARM					
CALF					
WEIGHT					

TOTAL WEIGHT LOSS >>

MONTHLY PROGRESS *Tracker*

JAN FEB MAR APR MAY JUN JUL AUG SEP OCT NOV DEC

MON	TUE	WED	THU	FRI	SAT	SUN

WEIGHT LOSS MILESTONE TRACKER

CHEAT DAY TRACKER

WEEKLY DIET SUCCESS TRACKER & NOTES

MY WEIGHT LOSS *Routine*

CREATING A ROUTINE FOR SUCCESS

WEIGHT LOSS SUCCESS: HABIT & ROUTINE TRACKER	
DRINK LOTS OF WATER TODAY	TRACK TOTAL CARB INTAKE

COMPLETE TOP 3 GOALS OF THE DAY

1.
2.
3.

PLAN MY MEALS FOR THE DAY:

BREAKFAST	LUNCH	DINNER

DAILY TRACKER & TO DO LIST	ACCOMPLISHMENTS

NOTES

My Routine

Morning   My Weight Loss Routine   m t w t f s s

Mid Day   My Weight Loss Routine   m t w t f s s

Evening   My Weight Loss Routine   m t w t f s s

Night   My Weight Loss Routine   m t w t f s s

WEEKLY *Fasting Tracker*

Week Of: _____

MONDAY

Goal 12 1 2 3 4 5 6 7 8 9 10 11 12 1 2 3 4 5 6 7 8 9 10 11

Actual 12 1 2 3 4 5 6 7 8 9 10 11 12 1 2 3 4 5 6 7 8 9 10 11

TUESDAY

Goal 12 1 2 3 4 5 6 7 8 9 10 11 12 1 2 3 4 5 6 7 8 9 10 11

Actual 12 1 2 3 4 5 6 7 8 9 10 11 12 1 2 3 4 5 6 7 8 9 10 11

WEDNESDAY

Goal 12 1 2 3 4 5 6 7 8 9 10 11 12 1 2 3 4 5 6 7 8 9 10 11

Actual 12 1 2 3 4 5 6 7 8 9 10 11 12 1 2 3 4 5 6 7 8 9 10 11

THURSDAY

Goal 12 1 2 3 4 5 6 7 8 9 10 11 12 1 2 3 4 5 6 7 8 9 10 11

Actual 12 1 2 3 4 5 6 7 8 9 10 11 12 1 2 3 4 5 6 7 8 9 10 11

FRIDAY

Goal 12 1 2 3 4 5 6 7 8 9 10 11 12 1 2 3 4 5 6 7 8 9 10 11

Actual 12 1 2 3 4 5 6 7 8 9 10 11 12 1 2 3 4 5 6 7 8 9 10 11

SATURDAY

Goal 12 1 2 3 4 5 6 7 8 9 10 11 12 1 2 3 4 5 6 7 8 9 10 11

Actual 12 1 2 3 4 5 6 7 8 9 10 11 12 1 2 3 4 5 6 7 8 9 10 11

SUNDAY

Goal 12 1 2 3 4 5 6 7 8 9 10 11 12 1 2 3 4 5 6 7 8 9 10 11

Actual 12 1 2 3 4 5 6 7 8 9 10 11 12 1 2 3 4 5 6 7 8 9 10 11

WEEK OF: *Meal* **LOG BOOK**

	BREAKFAST	LUNCH	DINNER	SNACKS
MONDAY				
TUESDAY				
WEDNESDAY				
THURSDAY				
FRIDAY				
SATURDAY				
SUNDAY				
	BREAKFAST	LUNCH	DINNER	SNACKS

MY PROGRESS *Tracker*

SLEEP TRACKER: DATE _____

 RISE: _____   BEDTIME: _____   SLEEP (HRS): _____

NOTES FOR THE DAY
_____
_____

IN A STATE OF KETOSIS?
YES   NO   UNSURE

WATER INTAKE TRACKER

EXERCISE / WORKOUT ROUTINE

DAILY ENERGY LEVEL		
HIGH	**MEDIUM**	**LOW**

BREAKFAST

FAT: CARBS: PROTEIN: CALORIES:

LUNCH

FAT: CARBS: PROTEIN: CALORIES:

DINNER

FAT: CARBS: PROTEIN: CALORIES:

SNACKS

FAT: CARBS: PROTEIN: CALORIES:

TOP 6 PRIORITIES OF THE DAY

END OF THE DAY TOTAL OVERVIEW

CARBS   FAT   PROTEIN   CALORIES

Macro Quick Reference

MACRO TRACKER

QTY	TYPE	PROTEIN	FAT	CARBS	CALS	NOTES

INTERMITTENT *Fasting Log*

WEEK OF:

	START TIME	END TIME	TOTAL FAST HRS
M	:	:	:
T	:	:	:
W	:	:	:
T	:	:	:
F	:	:	:
S	:	:	:
S	:	:	:

WEEK OF:

	START TIME	END TIME	TOTAL FAST HRS
M	:	:	:
T	:	:	:
W	:	:	:
T	:	:	:
F	:	:	:
S	:	:	:
S	:	:	:

WEEK OF:

	START TIME	END TIME	TOTAL FAST HRS
M	:	:	:
T	:	:	:
W	:	:	:
T	:	:	:
F	:	:	:
S	:	:	:
S	:	:	:

WEEK OF:

	START TIME	END TIME	TOTAL FAST HRS
M	:	:	:
T	:	:	:
W	:	:	:
T	:	:	:
F	:	:	:
S	:	:	:
S	:	:	:

WEEK OF:

	START TIME	END TIME	TOTAL FAST HRS
M	:	:	:
T	:	:	:
W	:	:	:
T	:	:	:
F	:	:	:
S	:	:	:
S	:	:	:

WEEK OF:

	START TIME	END TIME	TOTAL FAST HRS
M	:	:	:
T	:	:	:
W	:	:	:
T	:	:	:
F	:	:	:
S	:	:	:
S	:	:	:

MILESTONES & ACCOMPLISHMENTS

NOTES & REFLECTIONS

GOALS & *Accomplishments*

MONTH   JAN   FEB   MAR   APR   MAY   JUN   JUL   AUG   SEP   OCT   NOV   DEC

THIS MONTH'S **GOALS**

ACTION PLAN

M T W T F S S

NOTES:

WEEKLY GOALS

M
T
W
T
F
S
S

THOUGHTS

MEALS: | **BREAKFAST** | **LUNCH** | **DINNER** | **SNACKS**

M
T
W
T
F
S
S

Low Carb Shopping List

FRESH PRODUCE

MEAT AND SEAFOOD

DAIRY PRODUCTS

PANTRY ITEMS

FROZEN / OTHER

Friendly Foods

KETO FRIENDLY FOODS	NET CARBS	PROTEINS	FAT

FOODS TO EAT IN MODERATION	NET CARBS	PROTEINS	FAT

STAYING *On Track*

MY WEIGHT LOSS DIARY:

WATER TRACKER

LOW CARB SNACKS

NOTES & REMINDERS

DOODLE MY MOOD

BREAKFAST IDEAS

LUNCH IDEAS

DINNER IDEAS

STAYING *On Track*

MY WEIGHT LOSS DIARY:

WATER TRACKER

LOW CARB SNACKS

NOTES & REMINDERS

DOODLE MY MOOD

BREAKFAST IDEAS

LUNCH IDEAS

DINNER IDEAS

STAYING *On Track*

MY WEIGHT LOSS DIARY:

WATER TRACKER

LOW CARB SNACKS

NOTES & REMINDERS

DOODLE MY MOOD

BREAKFAST IDEAS

LUNCH IDEAS

DINNER IDEAS

STAYING *On Track*

MY WEIGHT LOSS DIARY:

WATER TRACKER

LOW CARB SNACKS

NOTES & REMINDERS

DOODLE MY MOOD

BREAKFAST IDEAS

LUNCH IDEAS

DINNER IDEAS

STAYING *On Track*

MY WEIGHT LOSS DIARY:

WATER TRACKER

LOW CARB SNACKS

NOTES & REMINDERS

DOODLE MY MOOD

BREAKFAST IDEAS

LUNCH IDEAS

DINNER IDEAS

STAYING *On Track*

MY WEIGHT LOSS DIARY:

WATER TRACKER

LOW CARB SNACKS

NOTES & REMINDERS

DOODLE MY MOOD

BREAKFAST IDEAS

LUNCH IDEAS

DINNER IDEAS

STAYING *On Track*

MY WEIGHT LOSS DIARY:

WATER TRACKER

LOW CARB SNACKS

NOTES & REMINDERS

DOODLE MY MOOD

BREAKFAST IDEAS

LUNCH IDEAS

DINNER IDEAS

MEAL *Planner*

WEEK OF

GROCERY LIST

MON

TUES

WED

THUR

FRI

SAT

SUN

My Recipes

RECIPE NAME:

Keto ☐ Low Carb ☐ Paleo ☐ Vegetarian ☐ Vegan ☐ Dairy Free ☐ Gluten Free ☐

QTY	INGREDIENTS	RECIPE INSTRUCTIONS

NOTES & RECIPE REVIEW

Serves	
Prep Time	
Cook Time	
Tools	
Temp	

Total	Carbs	Fat	Protein	Cals

DAILY FOOD *Tracker*

FOOD TRACKER

MEAL/SNACK	NET CARBS	FAT	CAL	PROTEIN
DAILY GOAL:				
TOTAL:				

NOTES & MEAL IDEAS

FITNESS TRACKER

		Notes
Type		
Time		
Avg HR		
Max HR		
Reps		
Cals		

DAILY OVERVIEW

		Notes		
Sleep			On Track	☐
Water Intake				
Steps Taken				
Active Mins			Goal Met	☐
Active Hours				
Cals Burned				

DAILY FOOD *Tracker*

FOOD TRACKER

MEAL/SNACK	NET CARBS	FAT	CAL	PROTEIN
DAILY GOAL:				
TOTAL:				

NOTES & MEAL IDEAS

FITNESS TRACKER

		Notes
Type		
Time		
Avg HR		
Max HR		
Reps		
Cals		

DAILY OVERVIEW

		Notes		
Sleep			On Track	☐
Water Intake				
Steps Taken				
Active Mins			Goal Met	☐
Active Hours				
Cals Burned				

DAILY FOOD *Tracker*

FOOD TRACKER

MEAL/SNACK	NET CARBS	FAT	CAL	PROTEIN
DAILY GOAL:				
TOTAL:				

NOTES & MEAL IDEAS

FITNESS TRACKER

- Type
- Time
- Avg HR
- Max HR
- Reps
- Cals

Notes

DAILY OVERVIEW

- Sleep
- Water Intake
- Steps Taken
- Active Mins
- Active Hours
- Cals Burned

Notes

On Track ☐

Goal Met ☐

DAILY FOOD *Tracker*

FOOD TRACKER

MEAL/SNACK	NET CARBS	FAT	CAL	PROTEIN
DAILY GOAL:				
TOTAL:				

NOTES & MEAL IDEAS

FITNESS TRACKER

		Notes
Type		
Time		
Avg HR		
Max HR		
Reps		
Cals		

DAILY OVERVIEW

		Notes		
Sleep			On Track	☐
Water Intake				
Steps Taken				
Active Mins			Goal Met	☐
Active Hours				
Cals Burned				

DAILY FOOD *Tracker*

FOOD TRACKER

MEAL/SNACK	NET CARBS	FAT	CAL	PROTEIN
DAILY GOAL:				
TOTAL:				

NOTES & MEAL IDEAS

FITNESS TRACKER

- Type
- Time
- Avg HR
- Max HR
- Reps
- Cals

Notes

DAILY OVERVIEW

- Sleep
- Water Intake
- Steps Taken
- Active Mins
- Active Hours
- Cals Burned

Notes

On Track ☐

Goal Met ☐

DAILY FOOD *Tracker*

FOOD TRACKER

MEAL/SNACK	NET CARBS	FAT	CAL	PROTEIN
DAILY GOAL:				
TOTAL:				

NOTES & MEAL IDEAS

FITNESS TRACKER

		Notes
Type		
Time		
Avg HR		
Max HR		
Reps		
Cals		

DAILY OVERVIEW

		Notes		
Sleep			On Track	☐
Water Intake				
Steps Taken				
Active Mins			Goal Met	☐
Active Hours				
Cals Burned				

DAILY FOOD *Tracker*

FOOD TRACKER

MEAL/SNACK	NET CARBS	FAT	CAL	PROTEIN
DAILY GOAL:				
TOTAL:				

NOTES & MEAL IDEAS

FITNESS TRACKER

- Type
- Time
- Avg HR
- Max HR
- Reps
- Cals

Notes

DAILY OVERVIEW

- Sleep
- Water Intake
- Steps Taken
- Active Mins
- Active Hours
- Cals Burned

Notes

On Track

Goal Met

GO TO *Meals*

FAVORITE AND FRIENDLY MEALS

BREAKFAST	LUNCH	DINNER	SNACKS
BREAKFAST	LUNCH	DINNER	SNACKS
BREAKFAST	LUNCH	DINNER	SNACKS
BREAKFAST	LUNCH	DINNER	SNACKS
BREAKFAST	LUNCH	DINNER	SNACKS
BREAKFAST	LUNCH	DINNER	SNACKS
BREAKFAST	LUNCH	DINNER	SNACKS

12 WEEK *Meal Tracker*

12 Week Challenge

MONTH	JAN	FEB	MAR	APR	MAY	JUN	JUL	AUG	SEP	OCT	NOV	DEC
WEEK	01	02	03	04	05	06	07	08	09	10	11	12

	BREAKFAST	LUNCH	DINNER	SNACKS
M				
T				
W				
T				
F				
S				
S				

GROCERY SHOPPING LIST / RECIPE INGREDIENTS

Weekly Meal Planner

Week of: _____

	Breakfast	Lunch	Dinner	Snack	Other
Monday	Carbs Fat Protein Cals TOTAL	Carbs Fat Protein Cals TOTAL	Carbs Fat Protein Cals TOTAL	Carbs Fat Protein Cals TOTAL	Carbs Fat Protein Cals TOTAL
Tuesday	Carbs Fat Protein Cals TOTAL	Carbs Fat Protein Cals TOTAL	Carbs Fat Protein Cals TOTAL	Carbs Fat Protein Cals TOTAL	Carbs Fat Protein Cals TOTAL
Wednesday	Carbs Fat Protein Cals TOTAL	Carbs Fat Protein Cals TOTAL	Carbs Fat Protein Cals TOTAL	Carbs Fat Protein Cals TOTAL	Carbs Fat Protein Cals TOTAL
Thursday	Carbs Fat Protein Cals TOTAL	Carbs Fat Protein Cals TOTAL	Carbs Fat Protein Cals TOTAL	Carbs Fat Protein Cals TOTAL	Carbs Fat Protein Cals TOTAL
Friday	Carbs Fat Protein Cals TOTAL	Carbs Fat Protein Cals TOTAL	Carbs Fat Protein Cals TOTAL	Carbs Fat Protein Cals TOTAL	Carbs Fat Protein Cals TOTAL
Saturday	Carbs Fat Protein Cals TOTAL	Carbs Fat Protein Cals TOTAL	Carbs Fat Protein Cals TOTAL	Carbs Fat Protein Cals TOTAL	Carbs Fat Protein Cals TOTAL
Sunday	Carbs Fat Protein Cals TOTAL	Carbs Fat Protein Cals TOTAL	Carbs Fat Protein Cals TOTAL	Carbs Fat Protein Cals TOTAL	Carbs Fat Protein Cals TOTAL

WEIGHT LOSS *Journal*

MONDAY

TUESDAY

WEDNESDAY

THURSDAY

FRIDAY

SATURDAY

SUNDAY

WEEK OF:

DATE	WEIGHT LOSS ACTION PLAN

NOTES

MY WEIGHT LOSS *Routine*

CREATING A ROUTINE FOR SUCCESS

WEIGHT LOSS SUCCESS: HABIT & ROUTINE TRACKER	
DRINK LOTS OF WATER TODAY	TRACK TOTAL CARB INTAKE

COMPLETE TOP 3 GOALS OF THE DAY

1
2
3

PLAN MY MEALS FOR THE DAY:

BREAKFAST	LUNCH	DINNER

DAILY TRACKER & TO DO LIST	ACCOMPLISHMENTS

NOTES

MY KETO *Routine*

Morning My Weight Loss Routine m t w t f s s

Mid Day My Weight Loss Routine m t w t f s s

Evening My Weight Loss Routine m t w t f s s

Night My Weight Loss Routine m t w t f s s

WEEKLY *Fasting Tracker*

Week Of: _____

MONDAY

Goal	12	1	2	3	4	5	6	7	8	9	10	11	12	1	2	3	4	5	6	7	8	9	10	11
Actual	12	1	2	3	4	5	6	7	8	9	10	11	12	1	2	3	4	5	6	7	8	9	10	11

TUESDAY

Goal	12	1	2	3	4	5	6	7	8	9	10	11	12	1	2	3	4	5	6	7	8	9	10	11
Actual	12	1	2	3	4	5	6	7	8	9	10	11	12	1	2	3	4	5	6	7	8	9	10	11

WEDNESDAY

Goal	12	1	2	3	4	5	6	7	8	9	10	11	12	1	2	3	4	5	6	7	8	9	10	11
Actual	12	1	2	3	4	5	6	7	8	9	10	11	12	1	2	3	4	5	6	7	8	9	10	11

THURSDAY

Goal	12	1	2	3	4	5	6	7	8	9	10	11	12	1	2	3	4	5	6	7	8	9	10	11
Actual	12	1	2	3	4	5	6	7	8	9	10	11	12	1	2	3	4	5	6	7	8	9	10	11

FRIDAY

Goal	12	1	2	3	4	5	6	7	8	9	10	11	12	1	2	3	4	5	6	7	8	9	10	11
Actual	12	1	2	3	4	5	6	7	8	9	10	11	12	1	2	3	4	5	6	7	8	9	10	11

SATURDAY

Goal	12	1	2	3	4	5	6	7	8	9	10	11	12	1	2	3	4	5	6	7	8	9	10	11
Actual	12	1	2	3	4	5	6	7	8	9	10	11	12	1	2	3	4	5	6	7	8	9	10	11

SUNDAY

Goal	12	1	2	3	4	5	6	7	8	9	10	11	12	1	2	3	4	5	6	7	8	9	10	11
Actual	12	1	2	3	4	5	6	7	8	9	10	11	12	1	2	3	4	5	6	7	8	9	10	11

WEEK OF: *Meal* **LOG BOOK**

	BREAKFAST	LUNCH	DINNER	SNACKS
MONDAY				
TUESDAY				
WEDNESDAY				
THURSDAY				
FRIDAY				
SATURDAY				
SUNDAY				

MY PROGRESS Tracker

SLEEP TRACKER: DATE

 RISE: BEDTIME: SLEEP (HRS):

NOTES FOR THE DAY

IN A STATE OF KETOSIS?

YES   NO   UNSURE

WATER INTAKE TRACKER

EXERCISE / WORKOUT ROUTINE

DAILY ENERGY LEVEL		
HIGH	**MEDIUM**	**LOW**

BREAKFAST

FAT: CARBS: PROTEIN: CALORIES:

LUNCH

FAT: CARBS: PROTEIN: CALORIES:

DINNER

FAT: CARBS: PROTEIN: CALORIES:

SNACKS

FAT: CARBS: PROTEIN: CALORIES:

TOP 6 PRIORITIES OF THE DAY

END OF THE DAY TOTAL OVERVIEW

CARBS   FAT   PROTEIN   CALORIES

Macro Quick Reference

MACRO TRACKER

QTY	TYPE	PROTEIN	FAT	CARBS	CALS	NOTES

QTY	TYPE	PROTEIN	FAT	CARBS	CALS	NOTES

INTERMITTENT Fasting Log

WEEK OF:

	START TIME	END TIME	TOTAL FAST HRS
M	:	:	:
T	:	:	:
W	:	:	:
T	:	:	:
F	:	:	:
S	:	:	:
S	:	:	:

WEEK OF:

	START TIME	END TIME	TOTAL FAST HRS
M	:	:	:
T	:	:	:
W	:	:	:
T	:	:	:
F	:	:	:
S	:	:	:
S	:	:	:

WEEK OF:

	START TIME	END TIME	TOTAL FAST HRS
M	:	:	:
T	:	:	:
W	:	:	:
T	:	:	:
F	:	:	:
S	:	:	:
S	:	:	:

WEEK OF:

	START TIME	END TIME	TOTAL FAST HRS
M	:	:	:
T	:	:	:
W	:	:	:
T	:	:	:
F	:	:	:
S	:	:	:
S	:	:	:

WEEK OF:

	START TIME	END TIME	TOTAL FAST HRS
M	:	:	:
T	:	:	:
W	:	:	:
T	:	:	:
F	:	:	:
S	:	:	:
S	:	:	:

WEEK OF:

	START TIME	END TIME	TOTAL FAST HRS
M	:	:	:
T	:	:	:
W	:	:	:
T	:	:	:
F	:	:	:
S	:	:	:
S	:	:	:

MILESTONES & ACCOMPLISHMENTS

NOTES & REFLECTIONS

GOALS &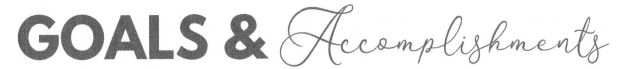

Month   JAN   FEB   MAR   APR   MAY   JUN   JUL   AUG   SEP   OCT   NOV   DEC

THIS MONTH'S **GOALS**

ACTION PLAN
M T W T F S S

NOTES:

WEEKLY GOALS
M
T
W
T
F
S
S

THOUGHTS

MEALS:	BREAKFAST	LUNCH	DINNER	SNACKS
M				
T				
W				
T				
F				
S				
S				

Low Carb Shopping List

FRESH PRODUCE

MEAT AND SEAFOOD

DAIRY PRODUCTS

PANTRY ITEMS

FROZEN / OTHER

Friendly Foods

KETO FRIENDLY FOODS	NET CARBS	PROTEINS	FAT

FOODS TO EAT IN MODERATION	NET CARBS	PROTEINS	FAT

STAYING *On Track*

MY WEIGHT LOSS DIARY:

WATER TRACKER

LOW CARB SNACKS

NOTES & REMINDERS

DOODLE MY MOOD

BREAKFAST IDEAS

LUNCH IDEAS

DINNER IDEAS

STAYING *On Track*

MY WEIGHT LOSS DIARY:

WATER TRACKER

LOW CARB SNACKS

NOTES & REMINDERS

DOODLE MY MOOD

BREAKFAST IDEAS

LUNCH IDEAS

DINNER IDEAS

STAYING *On Track*

MY WEIGHT LOSS DIARY:

WATER TRACKER

LOW CARB SNACKS

NOTES & REMINDERS

DOODLE MY MOOD

BREAKFAST IDEAS

LUNCH IDEAS

DINNER IDEAS

STAYING *On Track*

MY WEIGHT LOSS DIARY:

WATER TRACKER

LOW CARB SNACKS

NOTES & REMINDERS

DOODLE MY MOOD

BREAKFAST IDEAS

LUNCH IDEAS

DINNER IDEAS

STAYING *On Track*

MY WEIGHT LOSS DIARY:

WATER TRACKER

LOW CARB SNACKS

NOTES & REMINDERS

DOODLE MY MOOD

BREAKFAST IDEAS

LUNCH IDEAS

DINNER IDEAS

STAYING *On Track*

MY WEIGHT LOSS DIARY:

WATER TRACKER

LOW CARB SNACKS

NOTES & REMINDERS

DOODLE MY MOOD

BREAKFAST IDEAS

LUNCH IDEAS

DINNER IDEAS

STAYING *On Track*

MY WEIGHT LOSS DIARY:

WATER TRACKER

LOW CARB SNACKS

NOTES & REMINDERS

DOODLE MY MOOD

BREAKFAST IDEAS

LUNCH IDEAS

DINNER IDEAS

MEAL *Planner*

WEEK OF

GROCERY LIST

MON

TUES

WED

THUR

FRI

SAT

SUN

My Recipes

RECIPE NAME:

Keto ☐   Low Carb ☐   Paleo ☐   Vegetarian ☐   Vegan ☐   Dairy Free ☐   Gluten Free ☐

QTY	INGREDIENTS	RECIPE INSTRUCTIONS

NOTES & RECIPE REVIEW

Serves	
Prep Time	
Cook Time	
Tools	
Temp	

Total	Carbs	Fat	Protein	Cals

DAILY FOOD *Tracker*

FOOD TRACKER

MEAL/SNACK	NET CARBS	FAT	CAL	PROTEIN
DAILY GOAL:				
TOTAL:				

NOTES & MEAL IDEAS

FITNESS TRACKER

- Type
- Time
- Avg HR
- Max HR
- Reps
- Cals

Notes

DAILY OVERVIEW

- Sleep
- Water Intake
- Steps Taken
- Active Mins
- Active Hours
- Cals Burned

Notes

On Track

Goal Met

DAILY FOOD *Tracker*

FOOD TRACKER

MEAL/SNACK	NET CARBS	FAT	CAL	PROTEIN
DAILY GOAL:				
TOTAL:				

NOTES & MEAL IDEAS

FITNESS TRACKER

		Notes
Type		
Time		
Avg HR		
Max HR		
Reps		
Cals		

DAILY OVERVIEW

		Notes		
Sleep				On Track
Water Intake				
Steps Taken				
Active Mins				Goal Met
Active Hours				
Cals Burned				

DAILY FOOD *Tracker*

FOOD TRACKER

MEAL/SNACK	NET CARBS	FAT	CAL	PROTEIN
DAILY GOAL:				
TOTAL:				

NOTES & MEAL IDEAS

FITNESS TRACKER

		Notes
Type		
Time		
Avg HR		
Max HR		
Reps		
Cals		

DAILY OVERVIEW

		Notes		
Sleep			On Track	
Water Intake				
Steps Taken				
Active Mins			Goal Met	
Active Hours				
Cals Burned				

DAILY FOOD *Tracker*

FOOD TRACKER

MEAL/SNACK	NET CARBS	FAT	CAL	PROTEIN
DAILY GOAL:				
TOTAL:				

NOTES & MEAL IDEAS

FITNESS TRACKER

		Notes
Type		
Time		
Avg HR		
Max HR		
Reps		
Cals		

DAILY OVERVIEW

		Notes		
Sleep			On Track	☐
Water Intake				
Steps Taken				
Active Mins			Goal Met	☐
Active Hours				
Cals Burned				

DAILY FOOD *Tracker*

FOOD TRACKER

MEAL/SNACK	NET CARBS	FAT	CAL	PROTEIN
DAILY GOAL:				
TOTAL:				

NOTES & MEAL IDEAS

FITNESS TRACKER

- Type
- Time
- Avg HR
- Max HR
- Reps
- Cals

Notes

DAILY OVERVIEW

- Sleep
- Water Intake
- Steps Taken
- Active Mins
- Active Hours
- Cals Burned

Notes

On Track

Goal Met

DAILY FOOD *Tracker*

FOOD TRACKER

MEAL/SNACK	NET CARBS	FAT	CAL	PROTEIN
DAILY GOAL:				
TOTAL:				

NOTES & MEAL IDEAS

FITNESS TRACKER

		Notes
Type		
Time		
Avg HR		
Max HR		
Reps		
Cals		

DAILY OVERVIEW

		Notes		
Sleep			On Track	☐
Water Intake				
Steps Taken				
Active Mins			Goal Met	☐
Active Hours				
Cals Burned				

DAILY FOOD *Tracker*

FOOD TRACKER

MEAL/SNACK	NET CARBS	FAT	CAL	PROTEIN
DAILY GOAL:				
TOTAL:				

NOTES & MEAL IDEAS

FITNESS TRACKER

		Notes
Type		
Time		
Avg HR		
Max HR		
Reps		
Cals		

DAILY OVERVIEW

		Notes	
Sleep			On Track
Water Intake			
Steps Taken			
Active Mins			Goal Met
Active Hours			
Cals Burned			

GO TO Meals

FAVORITE AND FRIENDLY MEALS

BREAKFAST	LUNCH	DINNER	SNACKS
BREAKFAST	LUNCH	DINNER	SNACKS
BREAKFAST	LUNCH	DINNER	SNACKS
BREAKFAST	LUNCH	DINNER	SNACKS
BREAKFAST	LUNCH	DINNER	SNACKS
BREAKFAST	LUNCH	DINNER	SNACKS
BREAKFAST	LUNCH	DINNER	SNACKS

12 WEEK *Meal Tracker*

12 Week Challenge

MONTH	JAN	FEB	MAR	APR	MAY	JUN	JUL	AUG	SEP	OCT	NOV	DEC
WEEK	01	02	03	04	05	06	07	08	09	10	11	12

	BREAKFAST	LUNCH	DINNER	SNACKS
M				
T				
W				
T				
F				
S				
S				

GROCERY SHOPPING LIST / RECIPE INGREDIENTS

Weekly Meal Planner

Week of: _____

	Breakfast	Lunch	Dinner	Snack	Other
Monday	Carbs Fat Protein Cals TOTAL	Carbs Fat Protein Cals TOTAL	Carbs Fat Protein Cals TOTAL	Carbs Fat Protein Cals TOTAL	Carbs Fat Protein Cals TOTAL
Tuesday	Carbs Fat Protein Cals TOTAL	Carbs Fat Protein Cals TOTAL	Carbs Fat Protein Cals TOTAL	Carbs Fat Protein Cals TOTAL	Carbs Fat Protein Cals TOTAL
Wednesday	Carbs Fat Protein Cals TOTAL	Carbs Fat Protein Cals TOTAL	Carbs Fat Protein Cals TOTAL	Carbs Fat Protein Cals TOTAL	Carbs Fat Protein Cals TOTAL
Thursday	Carbs Fat Protein Cals TOTAL	Carbs Fat Protein Cals TOTAL	Carbs Fat Protein Cals TOTAL	Carbs Fat Protein Cals TOTAL	Carbs Fat Protein Cals TOTAL
Friday	Carbs Fat Protein Cals TOTAL	Carbs Fat Protein Cals TOTAL	Carbs Fat Protein Cals TOTAL	Carbs Fat Protein Cals TOTAL	Carbs Fat Protein Cals TOTAL
Saturday	Carbs Fat Protein Cals TOTAL	Carbs Fat Protein Cals TOTAL	Carbs Fat Protein Cals TOTAL	Carbs Fat Protein Cals TOTAL	Carbs Fat Protein Cals TOTAL
Sunday	Carbs Fat Protein Cals TOTAL	Carbs Fat Protein Cals TOTAL	Carbs Fat Protein Cals TOTAL	Carbs Fat Protein Cals TOTAL	Carbs Fat Protein Cals TOTAL

WEIGHT LOSS *Journal*

MONDAY

TUESDAY

WEDNESDAY

THURSDAY

FRIDAY

SATURDAY

SUNDAY

WEEK OF:

DATE	WEIGHT LOSS ACTION PLAN

NOTES

MY WEIGHT LOSS *Routine*

CREATING A ROUTINE FOR SUCCESS

WEIGHT LOSS SUCCESS: HABIT & ROUTINE TRACKER

DRINK LOTS OF WATER TODAY	TRACK TOTAL CARB INTAKE

COMPLETE TOP 3 GOALS OF THE DAY

1.
2.
3.

PLAN MY MEALS FOR THE DAY:

BREAKFAST	LUNCH	DINNER

DAILY TRACKER & TO DO LIST | ACCOMPLISHMENTS

NOTES

WEEKLY *Fasting Tracker*

Week Of: _____

MONDAY

Goal	12	1	2	3	4	5	6	7	8	9	10	11	12	1	2	3	4	5	6	7	8	9	10	11
Actual	12	1	2	3	4	5	6	7	8	9	10	11	12	1	2	3	4	5	6	7	8	9	10	11

TUESDAY

Goal	12	1	2	3	4	5	6	7	8	9	10	11	12	1	2	3	4	5	6	7	8	9	10	11
Actual	12	1	2	3	4	5	6	7	8	9	10	11	12	1	2	3	4	5	6	7	8	9	10	11

WEDNESDAY

Goal	12	1	2	3	4	5	6	7	8	9	10	11	12	1	2	3	4	5	6	7	8	9	10	11
Actual	12	1	2	3	4	5	6	7	8	9	10	11	12	1	2	3	4	5	6	7	8	9	10	11

THURSDAY

Goal	12	1	2	3	4	5	6	7	8	9	10	11	12	1	2	3	4	5	6	7	8	9	10	11
Actual	12	1	2	3	4	5	6	7	8	9	10	11	12	1	2	3	4	5	6	7	8	9	10	11

FRIDAY

Goal	12	1	2	3	4	5	6	7	8	9	10	11	12	1	2	3	4	5	6	7	8	9	10	11
Actual	12	1	2	3	4	5	6	7	8	9	10	11	12	1	2	3	4	5	6	7	8	9	10	11

SATURDAY

Goal	12	1	2	3	4	5	6	7	8	9	10	11	12	1	2	3	4	5	6	7	8	9	10	11
Actual	12	1	2	3	4	5	6	7	8	9	10	11	12	1	2	3	4	5	6	7	8	9	10	11

SUNDAY

Goal	12	1	2	3	4	5	6	7	8	9	10	11	12	1	2	3	4	5	6	7	8	9	10	11
Actual	12	1	2	3	4	5	6	7	8	9	10	11	12	1	2	3	4	5	6	7	8	9	10	11

WEEKLY *Progress*

WEEK OF : _____

Monday

Tuesday

Wednesday

Thursday

Friday

Saturday

Sunday

Notes

WEEK OF:

Meal LOG BOOK

	BREAKFAST	LUNCH	DINNER	SNACKS
MONDAY				
TUESDAY				
WEDNESDAY				
THURSDAY				
FRIDAY				
SATURDAY				
SUNDAY				
	BREAKFAST	LUNCH	DINNER	SNACKS

MY PROGRESS *Tracker*

SLEEP TRACKER:

DATE: _____

 RISE: _____   BEDTIME: _____   SLEEP (HRS): _____

NOTES FOR THE DAY
_____
_____

IN A STATE OF KETOSIS?

YES   NO   UNSURE

WATER INTAKE TRACKER

EXERCISE / WORKOUT ROUTINE

DAILY ENERGY LEVEL
HIGH   MEDIUM   LOW

BREAKFAST

FAT: CARBS: PROTEIN: CALORIES:

LUNCH

FAT: CARBS: PROTEIN: CALORIES:

DINNER

FAT: CARBS: PROTEIN: CALORIES:

SNACKS

FAT: CARBS: PROTEIN: CALORIES:

TOP 6 PRIORITIES OF THE DAY

END OF THE DAY TOTAL OVERVIEW

CARBS   FAT   PROTEIN   CALORIES

Notes

Notes

Notes

Made in the USA
Monee, IL
13 August 2023